Introduction to Pilates

I0417303

Use the Pilates Method to Get a Lean, Toned, Sexy Body

RON KNESS

ISBN-13: 978-1545133453

ISBN-10: 154513345X

Contents

Disclaimer

This publication is for informational purposes only and is not intended as medical advice. Medical advice should always be obtained from a qualified medical professional for any health conditions or symptoms associated with them.

Every possible effort has been made in preparing and researching this material. We make no warranties with respect to the accuracy, applicability of its contents or any omissions.

See your healthcare professional before starting any diet, health or exercise program!

Introduction

Pilates is a popular workout when you want to tone your body without weights or fancy gym equipment. It is something you can do anywhere, and very effective when you are consistent. It was originally invented by Joe Pilates, who wanted to help people align their spine, strengthen their core, and be aware of their muscles. Here are some things to know about Pilates.

What Pilates Does For Your Body

The first question you might be asking yourself is why you should do this type of workout. It is in fact similar to yoga, but it isn't the same thing nor should you have to choose one or the other. Yoga is great, but Pilates provides some unique benefits for your body and toning it.

Pilates moves really to work out your core, which is the primary reason to do the workout. It helps to flatten your tummy and strengthen your ab muscles. Then it also targets some other areas of your body, including 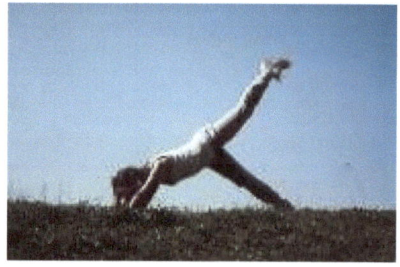 your legs, buttocks, arms, shoulders, and back.

You Can Do the Workout Anywhere

Another thing to know about Pilates is that while there are classes, you can easily do this right from home. There are videos found online, DVDs you can purchase, and even books that will provide images and descriptions of the different moves.

However, if you like to be in a community of others enjoying the same workout, you might like Pilates classes. The great thing about this workout is that you can travel and still do it right in your hotel room.

There Are Different Forms of Pilates

You will also notice that there are many different types of Pilates you can do. There is the classic form, with Joe Pilates' 23 basic moves. Plus contemporary Pilates mixing some different techniques, often including yoga or cardio workouts.

You may be interested in reformer Pilates, which uses a workout machines called a reformer. This moves your body in different ways, but provides more stability for the different workouts. Then there are specific types of Pilates like Power Pilates and Stott Pilates.

If you are interested in trying this workout, don't feel too pressured to get everything right the first time. It is working your core and strengthening your muscles, but it does take some practice. Some of the moves can be a little advanced, but the more you do them, the easier they become.

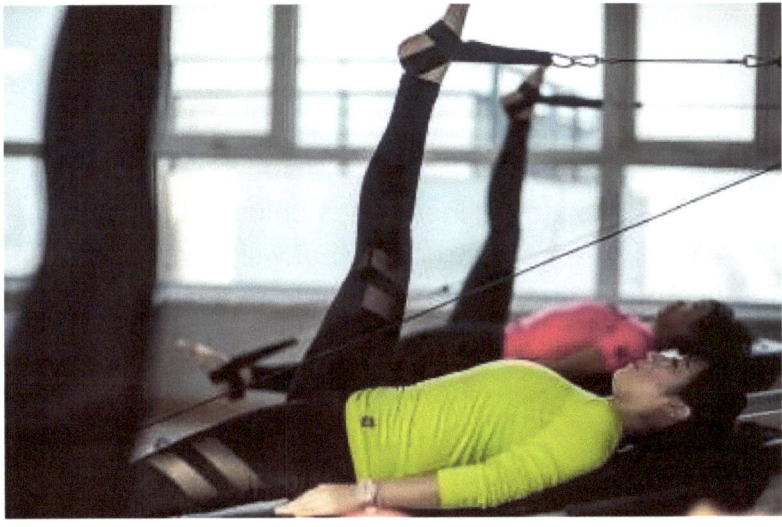

Types of Pilates

While the basic Pilates that Joe Pilates invented is still practiced today, there are many other forms as well. Here are some different types of Pilates to consider trying out.

Reformer Pilates

The first type of Pilates you can try out is called Reformer Pilates. This is a type of Pilates you do with a workout machine called a reformer. It has actually been around since the classic form of Pilates and was invented by Mr. Joseph Pilates himself.

The original reformer included a frame similar to a small bed with a flat platform that moved back and forth on the frame. This would help to do some different types of Pilates workouts, depending on where your body was positioned. There are newer versions of this same machine depending on where you get it and the types of Pilates moves you want to do.

Yoga-Pilates

This isn't just one type, but a concept based on different variations. There are fitness instructors online (Blogilates for example) as well as local instructors that will have a class where they combine yoga and Pilates into one workout.

This often includes some of the important core workout you learn in Pilates, helping to strengthen your abs and work on your core muscles, but also does a lot of the classic yoga moves mixed in as well. This helps to provide you with a solid

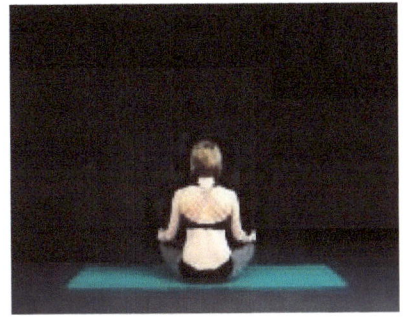

foundation and provide a good full-body workout.

Stott Pilates

You may also have heard of a type of Pilates called Stott Pilates. This form of Pilates was invented by a dancer, therefore it does include quite a few dancer moves and conditioning exercises along with Pilates. It uses some of the more modern workout moves with Pilates for a full-body workout.

Some other types of Pilates that you might hear about are Fletcher Pilates, Power Pilates, and Winsor Pilates. Then there are instructors at different fitness centers that have Pilates classes, but incorporate their own style and workout moves. It is good to try some different workouts until you find the one that works best for you.

Some do best with the original 23 classic Pilates moves, while others like to incorporate yoga, dance, or aerobic type workouts into their routine.

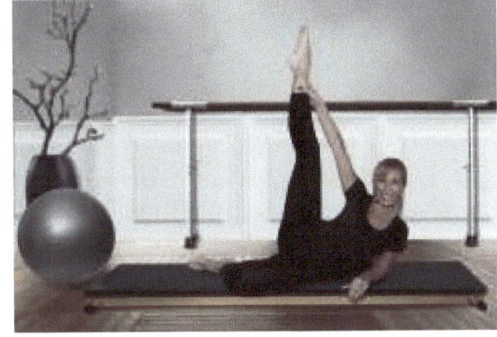

It isn't so much that you need to choose one, but that you should try different varieties until you find the workout that is perfect for you.

Benefits of Doing Pilates

If you are still on the fence about whether or not you should try Pilates, don't worry! There are a lot of health benefits, from fitness to non-fitness benefits. Here are some reasons you should try Pilates.

Get a Long, Fit Body

First of all, the reason why a lot of people turn to Pilates as their form of exercise is because it helps to create a long, lean, and strong body. You aren't going to bulk up with this exercise, but work on your core, strengthen your muscles, and really help to elongate your body. In the process, it is working on full-body muscle groups, and improving your balance, posture, and flexibility as well.

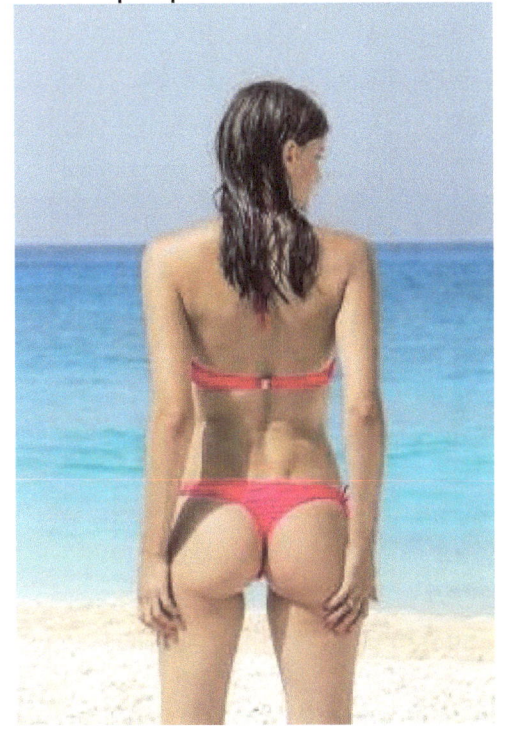

You Can Improve Your Memory

Not all benefits of doing Pilates are strictly for your body or getting toned. There are also mental benefits, including improving your memory. There have been studies done that show Pilates helps you to focus better, which in turn can improve your brain function and your memory capacity.

Even still, Pilates is a great way to start learning how to stop what you are doing and focus on the different movements, which is going to be a great benefit for you.

It is a Calming Experience

Pilates is often grouped with yoga because some of the moves are similar, and many of the benefits are the same. One of the same benefits is that Pilates helps to relax you and create a state of calm.

It is not a high-paced cardio workout or even a hard weight lifting workout. It is a slow, methodical exercise where you focus on your breathing, engage your core, and let your muscles do all the work.

You Can Get Abs

Going back to the physical aspects of Pilates is the fact that it helps to give you those abdominal muscles you have been wanting. Pilates goes far beyond just what crunches and sit-ups can do for you.

There are a lot of different movements that really strengthen your core, doing a lot of moves for flattening your tubby and even giving you some abs. It is going to work out your upper and lower abdominal muscles, as well as your obliques.

Give it a try for a month and see what a difference it has made in your abdomen. Plus, as an added bonus, your legs and arms get a good workout as well.

Best Moves for Beginners

Pilates is an effective workout, but not an easy one. It definitely takes practice with doing the moves and strengthening your muscles. However, there are some moves that are good for beginners to get you accustomed to the workout routine and start practicing the basics.

The Basic 100 Move

This isn't exactly the easiest move you will do in Pilates, but it is likely the first one you will learn. Even if you can only do Pilates for 5 minutes in the beginning, it should be the basic move.

The basic 100 move involves laying on your mat on your back, then bringing both legs close to your chest. You will hold onto them, curl your head up, then put your feet out like a tabletop. You will hold your arms to your sides and move them up and down for 100 quick reps. When just starting out, try to do about 20, then move to 50, then 100 if you need to.

The Abs Roll Up

This might go by different name, but it is another excellent Pilates move to strengthen your abdominal muscles, even when you are just starting out with this type of workout.

You will sit on your mat with your legs straight out in front of you, then move your body forward until your head is lowered close to your knees. Then move backward, but bend your knees and stop before you hit the ground. Raise your arms at this position and try to repeat multiple roll-up ab moves.

Single-Leg Tease Move

This type of move is going to work your legs and your core to get more muscles strengthened. It is good to start with this move before moving on to having both legs in the air at the same time. You will lie flat on the mat, with one leg extending out and one bent with your knee pointing up.

Reach forward as if trying to touch your toes, then roll down. Do a few reps of this, then alternate your legs and do it the same on the other side. Eventually, both of your legs will be pointed out while doing this move.

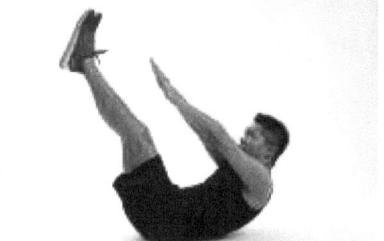

There are a lot of Pilates move that have similar modifications. These are going to help you to do Pilates even in the beginning, regardless of your experience, and soon become strong enough for the more advanced moves.

Best Beginner Pilates Tips

Are you interested in Pilates but haven't tried a workout yet? If so, the following tips can help get you started.

Use a Quality Pilates Mat

The mat you use does make a big difference because if you don't like how it feels or even how it looks, you are not as encouraged to keep up with your workouts. People often assume it doesn't matter what you workout in or with (like clothes or the mat), but it can  make a difference and actually make you excited to get started.

Since a lot of Pilates is done on the floor, you want to be as comfortable as possible with a really high-quality mat that is cushioned. Typical yoga mats is what you will look for, but make sure it is the right thickness.

Have Comfortable Clothing

The next thing you should make sure you have is comfortable clothing for the workouts. Since you are moving your body a lot in Pilates, try to avoid heavy 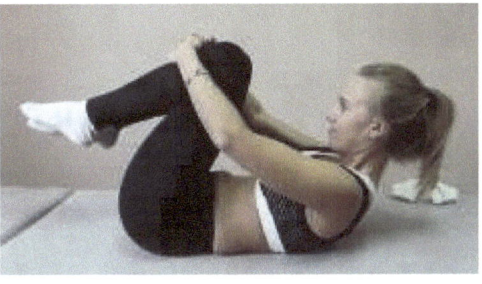 sweatpants that are difficult to move in or baggy t-shirts.

This can make some of the moves awkward.

You can usually do good with a fitted tee or tank top and yoga pants, but just pick something you are comfortable wearing for the Pilates class.

Remember that you will be barefoot, so don't worry about socks or shoes.

Take at Least One Pilates Class

There are different ways to start Pilates, from taking a local class to doing the exercises at home. However, even though watching YouTube videos or using a Pilates DVD is a convenient option, it is hard to learn the core moves properly 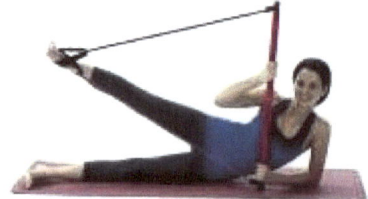 when you do it yourself. It is recommended that beginners at least take one or a few classes with an instructor to make sure you have the moves down.

Know What Your Body Can Handle

Pilates is not an exercise you will be able to do flawlessly and completely the first time you try it. The point is to strengthen your body gradually, so be patient and don't push too hard. If you can only do 5 reps of a new move instead of 10, do 5 and rest. The next time you try it, see if you can do 6, then 7 and so on until you hit those 10 reps.

If you need to modify some moves until you get stronger, don't be afraid to do so! Your body will eventually get stronger to where you don't need these adjustments.

Avoiding Common Pitfalls

As with most things, there are always errors that we should steer clear of when doing Pilates. Knowing what these errors are and rectifying them is crucial to getting the best from your workouts.

This chapter will list some of the most common mistakes that many people make when doing Pilates. Be mindful of them and correct yourself. You absolutely must be focused during your Pilates workout. This is how Pilates helps you to achieve the mind-body connection.

Not breathing correctly

A very common mistake. Beginners are so busy trying to execute the move correctly that they forget to match their inhaling and exhaling to their efforts. When you are easing up on a move, you inhale. When your exerting to execute a move, you exhale. Just remember – exhale when you exert.

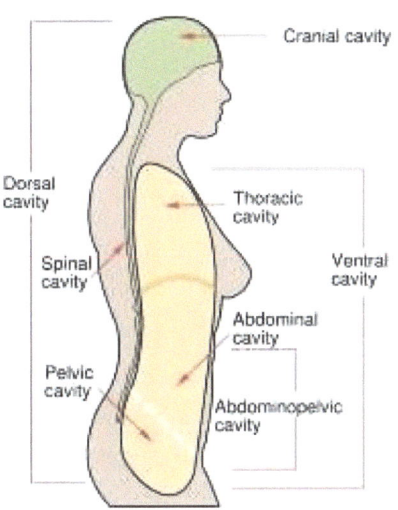

Not sucking in the abdominals

Pilates focuses most of its attention on your core. You're always told to suck in your navel towards your spine. This not only tones your core but creates a vacuum in your midsection that will give you a flatter tummy.

You must engage your core properly throughout the workout. It's common for people to relax the midsection after the first rep. This is wrong. You engage your core throughout the workout.

Rushing through the moves

People tend to believe that doing things faster equates to doing things better. While this may be true with other things, when it comes to Pilates, haste makes waste. You want to be slow and controlled. If you are rushing through the moves, your form will be compromised.

Another point to note is that Pilates becomes less challenging when you do the moves fast. Pilates uses isometric contraction to engage the muscles and make them work harder.

By rushing through the moves, the tension that is so beneficial to the muscles will be sacrificed.

Shoulders raised/Head hanging – Not in alignment

Your shoulders should always be flat and facing forward when doing moves that involve a plank position. Keeping your shoulders raised is a common mistake that must be avoided. Another mistake closely linked to this is hanging your head down instead of keeping it in alignment with your spine.

When doing moves such as the 'leg pull front' you will need to keep your shoulder down and facing forward and your head up. If you're tired and it's too difficult to keep your head up, do take a break. Never sacrifice form just to complete your workout.

It's better to stop your Pilates workout halfway if you're tired than to haphazardly do it just to say to say you completed it.

Lack of control/Too much momentum

Control is everything. Remember, Joseph even termed it 'contrology'. Don't be so focused on the external movements that you neglect the 'internal part' of the exercise. Ninety percent of Pilates' focus in internal.

So, keep your movements slow, steady… and most importantly, you MUST feel the movement when doing it.

You must feel the muscles working. Feel the fluidity, the resistance, the breathing – feel, feel, feel. This will keep you focused and your Pilates workouts will be fruitful.

Last but not least, do not fall into the trap of thinking that pain equals gain. Pilates can be challenging but you shouldn't force yourself and try to do too much too soon. You're trying to correct imbalances in your body, not create more.

There is no need to compete with your friends, other participants in the class, your spouse, etc. You just need to focus on yourself and make measurable progress in reasonable time. If you concern yourself with all the unnecessary distractions, you'll be taking away from your Pilates workouts and doing a disservice to yourself.

"Slow progress is better than no progress."

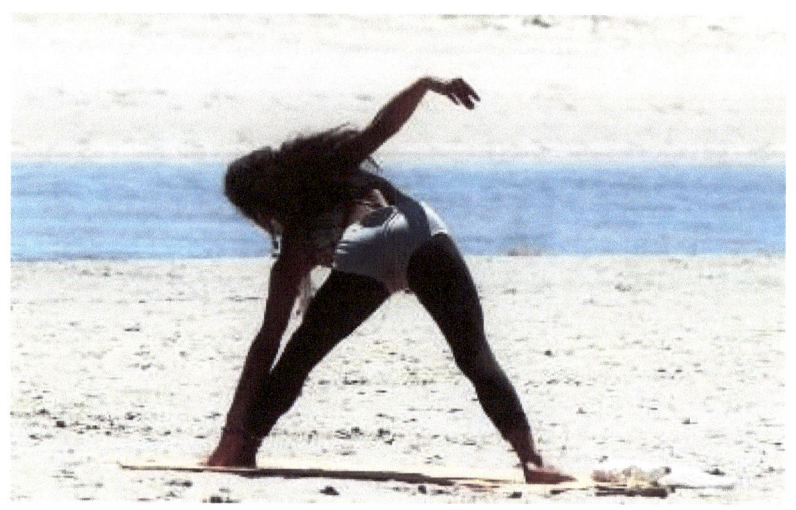

Accessories Used in Pilates

Pilates is an excellent exercise if you are looking to tone your muscles and increase flexibility. While Pilates focuses more on your core, many of the moves are also good for other areas of your body.

Pilates happens to be a workout that is often thought about as something you can do without any equipment, but there are actually quite a few accessories that would turn it into a full body workout. Here are some different accessories to consider using for your Pilates workout.

Exercise Balls

There are not one, but two different types of balls you can use with Pilates. The first is an exercise ball, sometimes referred to as a medicine ball. This type of ball is a larger size, and used for more types of exercises than just Pilates. You can use exercise balls in a number of different ways for your workouts, from leaning on the ball with your back and doing sit-ups for abs, to sitting on them in order to work on your balance and posture.

For Pilates, the exercise balls are used in various moves. You may fit the ball between your ankles and move your legs up as you move your upper body in a tight crunch that engages your core. There are standing and floor moves that is works great for.

The other type of ball you can use for your Pilates workouts is the mini ball. This is used specifically for Pilates and other similar workouts. It is smaller in size, up to about 9 inches in diameter.

You are able to use this ball for even more moves, making them a little more difficult and using more muscles with the ball.

Using a Ball For Pilates

Among the different accessories that can be used for Pilates, using a ball is a popular option. You can either use a medicine ball, also called an exercise ball, or a mini ball for a different set of exercises. Here are some ways to use a ball for Pilates.

Reach For the Stars

This Pilates move, often called a star reach, will actually provide more of a full-body workout. In addition to working on your abs and oblique muscles, it is also great for your legs and buttocks muscles. You are going to create a star-like shape with your entire body.

You will start with your feet apart, holding the ball in one hand. Lift the opposite leg to the side as high as you can, then bend your body to the opposite side and touch the ball to the floor. Keep that leg lifted as you bend, then go back up and repeat it. Don't forget to do the same amount of reps on the other side.

Work Your Triceps

This move is going to be for your triceps and shoulders, along with your abs like most Pilates workouts. It is a super easy way to use the ball for more of a workout.

For this move, you will lay down on your mat on one side, with that elbow touching the mat. The opposite arm is going to be up and out as you lift your body.

What you want to do is place the ball between your inner thighs, then raise the leg off the floor that is touching the mat, helping to lift your body.

Do Ball Pushups

This is a good option when you just want a super simple exercise by using the ball. Remember this is using a full-sized medicine ball, not the smaller Pilates balls.

For the ball pushups, you want to lay on top of the ball, with your abdomen touching it, then begin walking forward until you get the ball underneath where your thighs on. Now you can do pushups on the ground with the ball in this position. It helps to provide more stability for the move, while you engage your core and get a good arm workout at the same time.

Don't forget you can do a lot of different crunches by using the ball, depending on how you hold it. It is a great accessory to have for Pilates.

Foam Rollers

If you buy a Pilates package with multiple items to help with the workouts, it will likely include foam rollers. These are also used for different types of workouts, though many people prefer to use them for their Pilates workouts.

These rollers are made of soft or firm foam, are affordable, and help provide more stability for your different exercises. They can also be used to massage your tired and sore muscles after the Pilates workouts.

Foam Rolling Pilates Moves

One of the top accessories recommended for Pilates is the foam roller. This can also be used for other workouts, but people like to incorporate it into their daily core strengthening Pilates routine. Here are some moves you are able to do with the foam roller.

Ab and Hamstring Exercise

This first move that uses the Pilates foam roller is going to work both your core and your hamstrings, providing a good lower body workout. You will lay down with your stomach facing the mat, but put the foam roller under where your abdomen will be.

Bend your legs so that your heels can move up and work your glute muscles. Bring your arms back to take hold of your ankles and hold the position as long as you can, then release it. You can repeat this a few times until you feel a good burn.

Upper Body Foam Roller Move

The foam roller can also be used for some upper body Pilates-style moves. One of them is done by putting the foam roller underneath you while lying face-down on the mat, but this time it should be moved a little lower underneath your hips. You should be in a push up position where your upper torso meets the mat on the ground. Look up and arch your body until you feel your midsection and back start to stretch.

Another way to use it for an upper body workout is by sitting on the roller and place both hands behind you on the ground.

Arch your back, look up, and let your chest and upper arms get a good stretch.

Using the Roller For Classic Pilates

The foam roller can also just be used for the classic Pilates moves and exercises, not specific roller moves. Think of any moves you would do and how it can use a little more support from the foam roller. Perhaps you want to rest it underneath your knees so that extending your legs out is still a good workout, but not quite as difficult.

This would be really good to do when you are first starting out, because your abs are still being worked, but you have that extra support underneath your legs. Then when you feel comfortable doing so, remove the roller and do the entire Pilates exercise.

Keep the roller close to your Pilates mat during each session so you can grab it as needed.

Pilates Ring

There is also a Pilates ring, sometimes called a magic ring. This is a large ring that is a little flexible, but mostly a solid piece of equipment. You can hold it between your ankles as you move your legs up and down to work on your abdominal muscles, or lay on your side with the ring between your legs to do various exercises.

What Is a Pilates Reformer?

One of the types of Pilates is called reformer Pilates. This uses a workout machine designed specifically for the type of movements you would do in classic, mat Pilates. It provides more stability and a different set of workouts as well.

The Pilates Reformer

The Pilates reformer is a piece of workout equipment that looks similar to a rowing machine, but a little different. Instead of having a seat you sit in, there is a flat platform on top that you position yourself on in different ways, moving forward 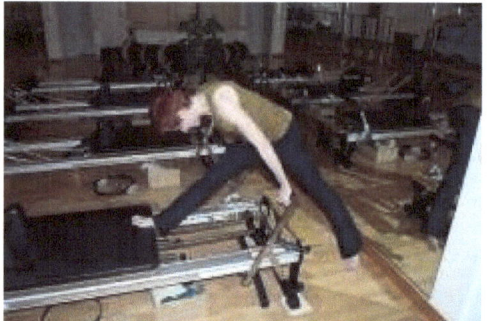 and backward for various Pilates moves.

The reformer was invented by Joseph Pilates shortly after he came up with the concept of Pilates for strength and flexibility, but it has gone through some variations since that first invention. You can find them on Amazon and stores selling sporting equipment, as well as some classes specifically for Reformer Pilates.

Why You Should Use a Reformer

You definitely don't have to get a reformer just to have a good Pilates workout, but it helps in a variety of ways. First of all, the machine provides more versatility in your movements.

Regular Pilates uses no equipment, but there are some moves you can't really do without pushing, pulling, or holding onto something.

This, among many other things, is where the reformer comes in. It allows you to try different moves in different angles, work a different muscle group, and simply make your Pilates workout more interesting.

Ways to Use the Pilates Reformer

There are actually a lot of different ways you can use a Pilates reformer. It just depends on how your body is positioned on the workout equipment. There is a foot bar, straps, and shoulder blocks, plus the flat platform.

You can do this in different positions like laying down on the platform, standing on it, sitting straight or at an angle, pushing the foot bar, using the foot bar to stand or sit, using other equipment, doing it upside down, and so many other unique ways. It looks like a simple piece of equipment, but there is a lot you can do with it.

If you want to learn how to use this type of machine, taking a class is your best option. The instructor will show you different things you can do with a reformer and provide a really fun class at the same time.

Final Thoughts - Making Pilates Part of Your Lifestyle

"We first make our habits, then our habits make us."

John Dryden

In order for you to truly benefit from Pilates, you must be consistent in your workouts. Fix a time each day when you'll do your Pilates session. Pilates is a gentle enough exercise for you to do daily.

In the event that you have muscular aches and pains from a previous session, you may take a break for a day or two. But you must get back on track. You MUST develop the habit of daily exercise.

Then, and only then, will you reap the full benefits of Pilates. It must become an integral part of your healthy lifestyle and not an afterthought.

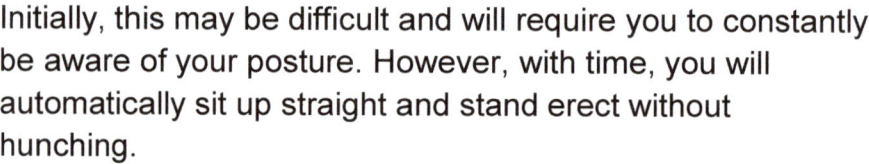

Besides regular sessions, you must also remember to maintain good posture throughout the day.

Initially, this may be difficult and will require you to constantly be aware of your posture. However, with time, you will automatically sit up straight and stand erect without hunching.

No exercise program is complete without some mention about your diet. Regardless of age, it would be a good idea to consume more vegetables and fruit. These are rich in antioxidants and beneficial nutrients. Eat in moderation and avoid processed foods.

It would be a good idea to slowly try and lose all excess weight. A simple 500-calorie per day deficit will slowly get rid of all the excess fat. Besides your Pilates session, you may wish to go for a 20 to 30-minute walk to get some sunshine and cardio activity.

Do not stress yourself over small things. They often say that, "It's not what you eat that makes you sick. It's what's eating you." To a large extent this is true. While a poor diet is to be avoided at all costs, being stress-free is just as important.

Pilates sessions are excellent for de-stressing because you will need to focus on the exercises and this will give you a mental break from your worries. Good health requires you to sweat the body and not the small stuff.

Last but not least, make sure you get enough rest and quality sleep. Pilates has been shown to promote better sleep since your muscles will be fatigued after the workouts and you will crave sleep.

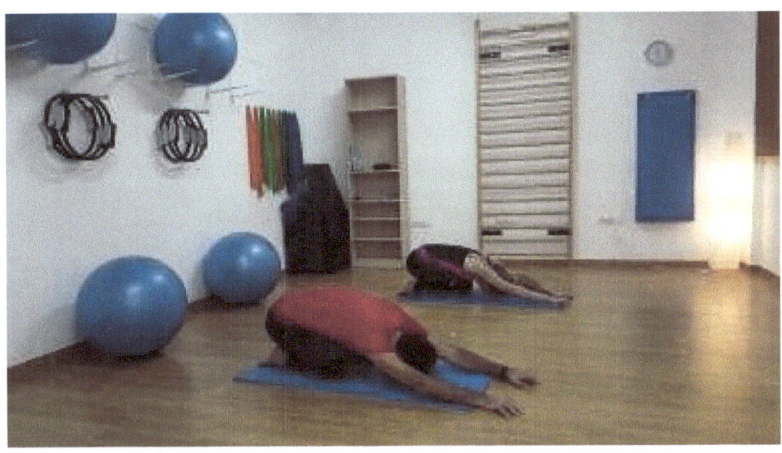

Resources

Listed below are some Amazon links to the various accessories referenced in this book that can be used in Pilates.

Reformer

http://amzn.to/2nuXqCl

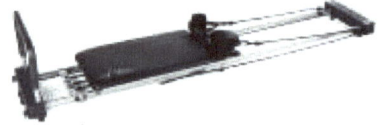

Mat

http://amzn.to/2ov3GLO

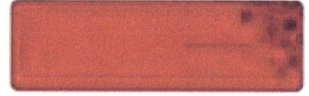

Ball

http://amzn.to/2mZR426

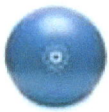

Pilates Ring

http://amzn.to/2mZBWBH

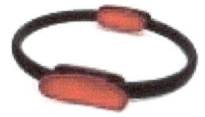

Resistance Band Set

http://amzn.to/2ouPm5M

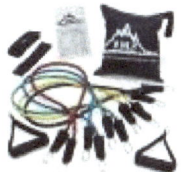

Exercise Ball Set

http://amzn.to/2mZKjNQ

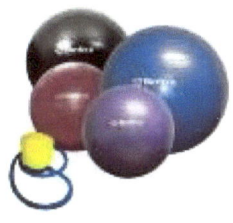

Other Relevant Books by This Author

If you would like to read more relevant books about this topic, here is a list of the CreateSpace links, titles and descriptions from this author:

https://www.createspace.com/7020067

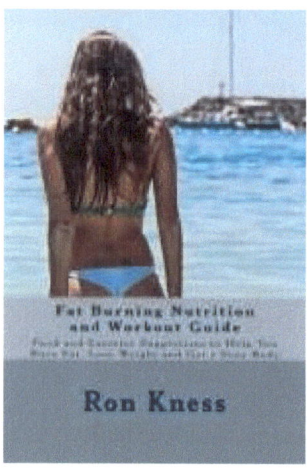

Fat Burning Nutrition and Workout Guide: Food and Exercise Suggestions to Help You Burn Fat, Lose Weight and Get a Sexy Body

We want to be more in charge of our weight loss efforts. We also want to find a program that works and one we can stay on indefinitely. And we want to eat foods and do exercise workouts that help burn fat!

We can achieve ALL of these goals with the newest release from Ron Kness called "Fat Burning Nutrition And Workout Guide".

Based on these exciting teachings, you will learn about all the dramatic benefits of eating healthy and working out as a way of burning fat to lose weight and why some workouts help burn fat better than others.

This book is built around a very clear, concept: burn fat, lose weight, and get a sexy body.

It's not just about losing weight. Having great eating habits is linked to better health too.

In this book, we look at ways you can improve your own eating habits, starting with portion control and food choices. This book will also look at the many other steps that can be taken to support this goal, from reading this guide, to following the advice in it on eating and working out. The choices you make today about food and exercising have a direct impact on your health tomorrow.

In "Fat Burning Nutrition And Workout Guide", we'll cover all the bases, giving you everything you need to know to maximize your weight loss efforts through the burning of fat.

https://www.createspace.com/6988390

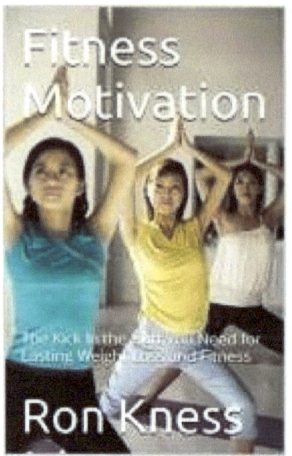

Fitness Motivation: The Kick In the Butt You Need for Lasting Weight Loss and Fitness

We want to be better about ourselves. We also want to be in control of our weight loss and fitness program. And we want to overcome adversity and negativity when on a weight loss and fitness program!

We can achieve ALL of these goals with the newest release from Ron Kness called "Fitness Motivation". Based on these exciting teachings, you will learn about all the dramatic benefits of staying the course when on a weight loss and fitness program and the immense value of having a positive mindset and eliminating negativity when trying to get fit.

This book is built around a very clear, concept: ultimately improve your body image through weight loss and fitness.

It's not just about learning to like yourself the way you are, although that can be hard in itself. Having great body image and high self-esteem is linked to being in charge of your own thinking. This is in part because you refuse to give in to body shaming and remove it from your life when possible.

In this book, we look at many different ways you can improve your own self-body image and self-esteem, starting with getting rid of negativity in your life. If that means dissolving some friendships that have a negative impact on you, then so be it!

This book will also look at the many other steps that can be taken to support this goal, from first determining what is causing adversity and negativity in your life to eliminating and replacing it with positivity. Even the choices you make about diet rewards and penalties can have an impact on your body image and self-esteem.

In "Fitness Motivation", we'll cover all the bases, giving you everything you need to know to stay motivated, learn from past failures, and to lose weight and get in great shape!

https://www.createspace.com/6923372

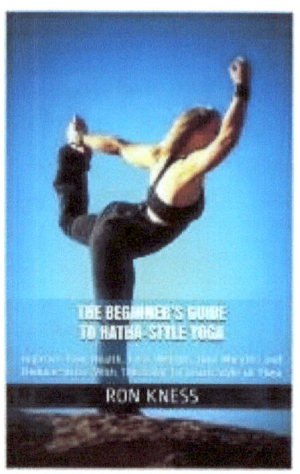

The Beginner's Guide to Hatha-Style Yoga: Improve Your Health, Lose Weight, Tone Muscles and Reduce Stress With This Easy-To-Learn Style of Yoga

We want there to be a calmness of in both our mind and spirit. We also want to be healthier as we age. And to accomplish both, we must learn to do the poses of Hatha yoga!

We can achieve ALL of these goals with the newest release from Ron Kness called "The Beginner's Guide To Hatha-Style Yoga".

Based on these exciting teachings, you will learn about all the dramatic benefits of doing Hatha yoga like improved health, weight loss, muscle toning and reducing stress, along with improved flexibility and balance.

This book is built around a very clear, concept: learn yoga and reap the benefits from doing this style of yoga - Hatha.

It's not just about learning how to do this easy-to-learn style of yoga. Having great overall health is linked to being in charge and making smart healthy lifestyle decisions. This is because learning how to do any style of yoga should be part of any healthy lifestyle.

In this book, we look at all of the ways you can improve your own overall health, starting with deciding to learn the poses and practice yoga. This book will also look at the many other steps that can be taken to support this goal, like viewing the suggested videos of poses used in Hatha yoga depending on the health benefit you want to gain.

The choices you make about joining a Hatha yoga class or learning it by yourself and doing it at home has a great impact on your overall health.

In "The Beginner's Guide To Hatha-Style Yoga", we'll cover all the bases, giving you everything you need to know to do this style of yoga that provides the health benefits mentioned.

Get your copy now and start improving your health tomorrow!

About the Author

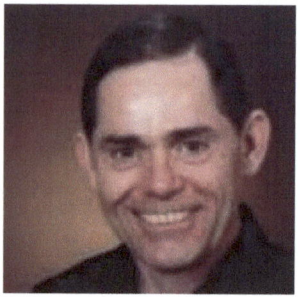

I have published over 125 books on Amazon for Kindle, CreateSpace and other publishing platforms.

While most of my books are on health and fitness in general, as I age (now 65) at the time of this writing) my topics of interest are geared toward aging baby boomers and older.

Besides my own writing, I also ghostwrite ebooks, books, reports, articles, blogs and do Kindle conversions for clients on a variety of topics.

Today my wife and I are retired from our careers and live in Gold Canyon, AZ. I now write as a retirement business where you'll find me happily sitting in my office typing away on my laptop as I work on my next book or ghostwriting project . . . that is if we are not traveling on a cruise ship - our new-found mode of travel.

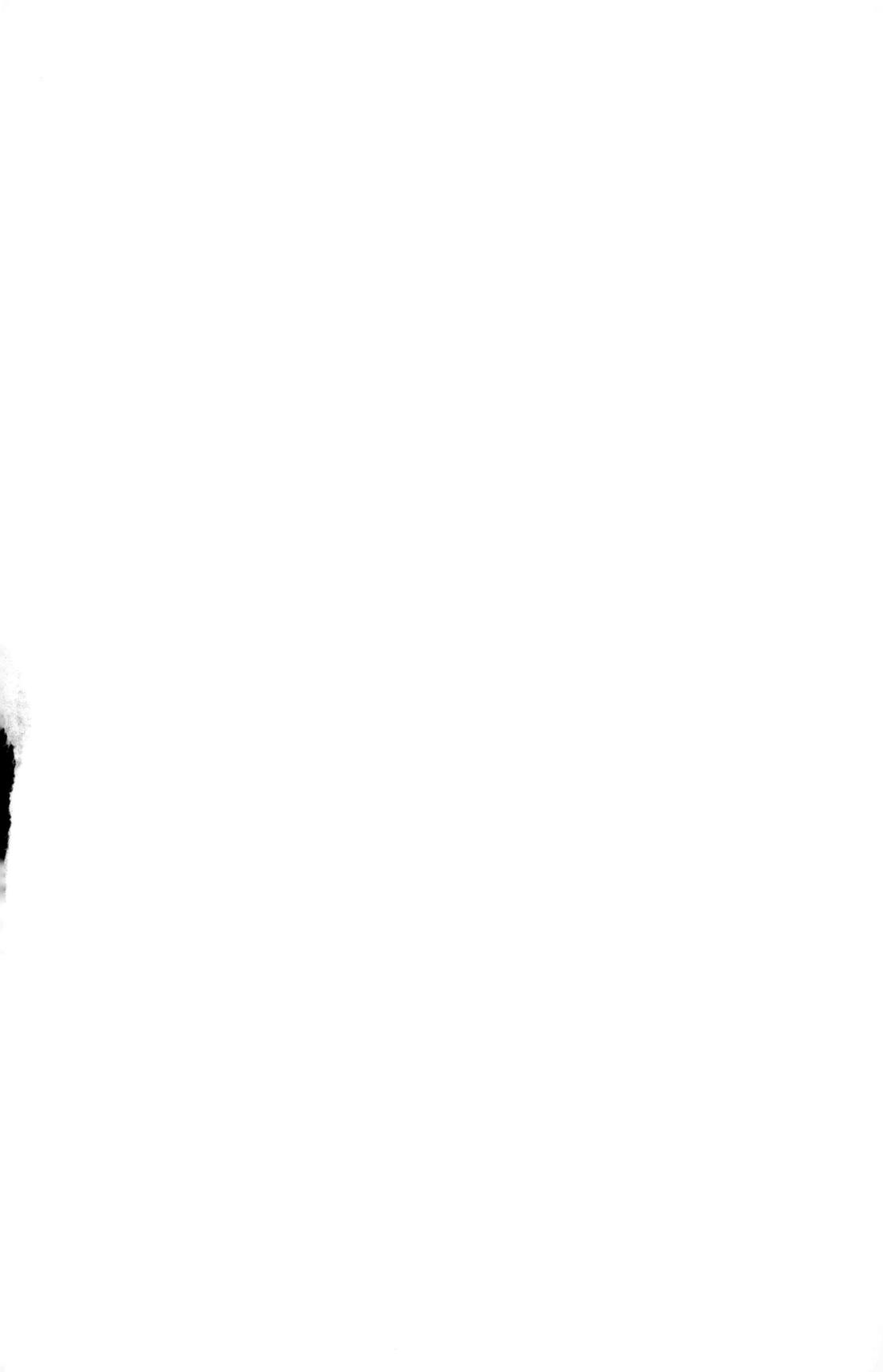

www.ingramcontent.com/pod-product-compliance
Lightning Source LLC
Chambersburg PA
CBHW050856290526
45792CB00002B/612